Gluten Free Living

A Dietary Lifestyle

By

Sally Parker

Here are a few more of my other books

HOW TO HAVE A SUCCESSFUL GARAGE SALE

SELLING GOODWILL ITEMS ON EBAY

You can also go to my Amazon Author page

Table of Contents

Introduction

If you know what gluten is, where it originates, and how to determine whether a food is likely to contain it, you are miles ahead in your thinking. The choice to go "gluten –free" is not easy, nor is it an easy decision to make in the first place.

This book is designed with the dietary-conscious in mind. If you picked it up because you are familiar with the subject, great! While it is true that only a small portion of the population have difficulty digesting the doughy, sticky protein that makes up a majority of the grains we eat on a daily basis, there is some merit in considering a diet free of it for more than simply its health concerns. This book attempts to demystify its challenges, and offers up a means to make such a dietary choice more one of understanding and awareness than fear and ignorance.

Medically, there are a small portion of the population that is absolutely negatively impacted by the existence of Gluten in their diets. Medically this group includes several characteristics and diseases that depend on the removal of gluten from the diet, and this book outlines those dangers and how best to live a gluten-free life.

For the most part, gluten is a protein found in predominately in the domesticated grains that we count as staples in our daily diet. Its positive qualities give breads, pastries, and cakes their pleasing elasticity. It helps these doughs to rise and keep shape, and offers the products made with these grains a chewy texture. These characteristics mean that it is found in a wide variety of food and healthcare products. While rice and some forms of maize (corn) have stored proteins that are also called glutens, these do not have the adverse allergic reactions, and therefore provide the means to have a virtually gluten-free diet as necessary.

What this book seeks to identify are the merits of a transition to this new kind of diet, and expresses the benefits – and the dangers – of making such a life-changing shift in your eating habits. We hope to educate and entertain you, and perhaps help you make a life-altering change in your eating habits.

We will cover the case against gluten, why is this so reviled, and what merit changing your diet to eliminate it may have. We'll go over the alternatives and substitutions one can make to keep a modicum of familiarity in their diet, and we will discuss briefly the challenge of understanding the vagaries of food labeling associated with cutting back on gluten.

Then we will talk about the non-medical reasons some offer to avoid glutens, as well as developing a moderated stance on food experimentation, leading to the full-on avoidance of gluten in one's diet.

Finally, we will talk about how to make the Gluten-free diet a reality, and how to achieve this goal, even while traveling or away from your home. We'll wrap up with some simple do's and don'ts in keeping a Gluten-Free Lifestyle, and conclude with some final notes on how to live with the benefits and the dangers of dealing with Celiac's disease and other grain intolerances.

1: The Case Against Gluten

The conversations across the internet about diet and health have been ablaze with proponents of and opposition to the growing interest in a Gluten-Free diet. The question that drives this controversy falls to a very basic concept: what is gluten, where does it come from, and why should anyone care?

The Gluten conversation actually begins with a disease that has been tracked and identified among the population, whose victims suffer digestion problems when eating breads, pastas, and doughs made from wheat, oats, barley, and other grains.

The disease commonly called Celiac's disease has been traced back over two thousand years, through study of the remains of persons who exhibited symptoms. It wasn't until the late 1880's, though, that it was associated with dietary issues, by Dr. Samuel Gee. His research on persons exhibiting the symptoms concluded that dietary changes could mitigate or alleviate altogether the symptoms, provided the amount to fried-dough foods were drastically reduced.

In this chapter, you will learn:

- The origins of awareness to the impact of gluten in medical knowledge

- The benefits to those impacted by the medical merits of a gluten-free diet

The Side Effects of Gluten Ingestion for sufferers of Celiac's

The sufferers of Celiac's disease have a real problem. The impact of a diet that includes gluten is damage to the small intestine which prevents the victim from getting proper nutrition through the small intestine, and leading to malnutrition, despite adequate food supply and quality. Although gluten is a cause for adverse reactions in people with Celiac's disease, it rarely impacts the digestion of others in any way. In the overall population, therefore, the amount of gluten has no effect whatsoever. As a comparative number only one in 133, or about one percent of Americans has diagnosable Celiac's disease, and only four percent have a specific wheat allergy. An even smaller percentage of Americans report any form of gluten intolerance, citing digestive problems that may or may not be related to the disease itself.

For comparison, 17% of Americans smoke today, compared to 20% as recently as 2005.

As Celiac's is an autoimmune disease, and not just a lifestyle choice, it is best to include your medical resources before changing your diet. The treatment of symptoms of this nature should be under the recommendation and awareness of your Doctor, and is a very serious part of your everyday health. If you do have Celiac's, these are the kinds of symptoms you will manifest if you eat Gluten, and are indeed a sufferer.

Symptoms of Celiac's

As with any internal organ issues, the sufferers of Celiac's experience a wide array of symptoms. Only medical practitioners can be certain of the presence of the disorder, but symptoms generally include fatigue, arthritis, constipation or loose stools, bone or joint discomfort, and many more. It is this generally indistinguishable set of symptoms that are the reason your medical team are best suited for determining whether or not you are a Celiac's sufferer. This applies as well to children, as they may have many sources for the symptoms as well.

Associated Syndromes and General Intolerance

Despite the lack of medical necessity, people may still choose to restrict or limit access to gluten for their own diet, for a myriad of reasons, none of which are of medical necessity. If you do choose to alter your diet, it is still greatly advised for you to contact and consult your medical authorities, to ensure your diet choices do not endanger your health in other, unforeseen ways. **Be aware that there are no positively affirmed benefits of a Gluten-free lifestyle, and that it is a mere personal choice, if not expressly defined by a medical authority.**

The Gluten-Free Lifestyle

As with any diet regimen, the choice to live without glutens in your meals requires discipline. For those whose choice is one of survival, of avoiding the dangers of Glutens when you suffer from Celiac's, the discipline is backed with the danger, and therefore perhaps a little easier to maintain. Still, the very nature of a restrictive diet can sometimes leave the participant with a longing for what they cannot have. In the case of a gluten-free existence, perhaps it is a bit easier, as the sources are fairly limited. Of course, staying away from breads, pastas, cereals and more, all of which have permeated and infused our diets since childhood is considerably more challenging than simply stating the desire to do so. This choice is, as with any other, a measured decision to do battle with our own desires and wants, in favor of what is best for our life, what is going to keep us alive.

2: Sources of and Alternatives to Gluten

Gluten in Everyday Life

Gluten, a naturally-formed protein found in most food sources that are associated with grains such as wheat, barley, oats and more, is of its own a food material that is defined by the Food and Drug Administration as generally regarded as safe (GRAS) foodstuff that does not require any particular labeling or categorization. Because of the attention that the substance has drawn recently, there are a variety of advertising and marketing ploys that play off the fears and concerns of those impacted by allergies, diseases, and bodily intolerance to it.

In this chapter, you will learn:

- Where gluten comes from, and how it gets into our diet

- Food alternatives that do not have the dangerous forms of gluten.

Sources of Gluten in American Diets

Nearly all forms of bread that is produced in the US and Canada had Gluten in it, though not specifically identified as such. Breads, rolls, biscuits, cookies, or other food materials made from wheat, rye, barley, or certain other grains are permeated with the stuff. As are virtually every cereal, cracker, and the like made from these same grains. Food stuffs like dried-bread stuffing, croutons, etc. that are derivatives of them, even soup stock or other byproducts of the grain category have loads of gluten in their composition. The good news is that in general, if you can avoid the grains that are the source, you will avoid most gluten resources.

The primary challenge, though, are those food sources that use these staples, but do not list them explicitly in the ingredients list. Many staples in processed forms, such as soups, frozen meals, and the like have added gluten for substance, making the search for gluten-free foods more challenging.

Dietary Replacements for Gluten Sources

Many other sources of dietary fiber do not have this particular protein configuration, so a person who adheres to a gluten-free diet is not restricted from being just as satisfied with other sources. In particular, the replacement for wheat, oats, and barley can include any or all of the following alternatives.

The list is actually compelling, if not as appetizing as they might be. Though unfamiliar with most American consumers, Amaranth, Quinoa, as well as Buckwheat groats, Millet, all viable grain replacements. More familiar, both Brown and Wild rice are known to be free of the dangerous form of gluten.. Certain Oats can also be used, but those you would want to go over with your doctor.

Granted, these grains are not as easily milled or used as the more common wheat, barley, or oats that are in common use. Fortunately, these are still quite accessible, particularly in large population centers. Natural food centers and farm communities are both great resources for such, and in certain communities, these can even be found in a flour-like form for direct substitution.

Changing the way we eat

Sandwiches, pizzas, even burritos, some of the most common foods in the American diet, are absolute dens of iniquity, from a gluten standpoint. All of the various types of bread that we eat are sources for the stuff, and while certain kinds of grains can be milled and used in the same fashion, it simply is not common fare, and usually requires one to prepare the bread themselves.

An easier way to eliminate or at least considerably reduce the gluten content, is to simply cease seeing these vehicles as the primary method to prepare food. Look to salads and barbecue as the new normal, with fresh meat and sautéed vegetables and such as common meal choices. When it comes down to it, the Paleo diet is not too far removed from one that is gluten-free, as both disdain processed foods in favor of fresh fruit, vegetables, and meats. Even the low-carb diets like South Beach and Atkins turn away from the processed breads and pastas, so there are many alternatives that can satify and keep the heart and mind engaged, thinking not about what is restricted, but rather about what is allowed.

Taking the time to shop daily, instead of buying in advance in bulk is another life change that can positively affect a gluten-free lifestyle. Simple foods, simply prepared – that will be the new normal. Keeping the eye on the prize, watching food labels and marketing ploys, will keep you and your family healthy and away from the dangers of Gluten.

3: Defining and Labeling Gluten-Free products.

Generally speaking, if you are talking about fresh food, straight from the garden, grown from the land and not processed like most foods you can purchase at a grocer's you won't find them to be sources of Gluten. Most folks, even if they are green thumbs and love to grow their own food, don't go so far as raising and milling their own flour from the land.

Indeed, it is when one supplements their diet with processed foods that issues of whether a food is gluten free comes up at all. This book will help take the mystery out of shopping for a gluten-free life.

In this chapter, you will learn:

- Distinctions in labeling, from voluntary to compulsory

- The appeal of Gluten-free, and how marketing takes advantage.

Understanding Gluten terms in Food Packaging and Production

As the natural foods that include gluten are well-known, it is primarily processed, packaged foods that are difficult to discern. Many have at least some gluten added for one reason or another, and therefore require laborious study, in order to protect one's self. These labels can be misleading or even untrue, so here are some Label Guidelines:

In order for a food to be allowed to call itself "Gluten Free", the foodstuff must contain no more than 20 parts per million. This is a rather significant level to attain, and the testing can be rather rigorous to achieve this distinction. As this has a testable limit, it is a fairly safe label to adhere to, compared with other more ambiguous terms.

A product may claim such neutral and seemingly benign terms as 'reduced gluten' or 'less gluten', but without qualifiers as to exactly how the Gluten was reduced, or compared to what measure they are considering it less than, these terms are misleading, and have no established veracity. Use these products carefully, or avoid them completely to be safe.

A more honest qualifier, such as "May contain Gluten" means that the process or production method that is employed to make the product may actually parallel that of known gluten-laden products. Therefore, the label is actually making no claim of being 'gluten free'. While this label may be misleading, it is at least acknowledging that the possibility exists that it may contain the substance, and thusly, they cannot use the more stringent label.

Be sure to confirm the status if gluten is a medical issue for you. If it is more philosophic, the secondary labeling will more than likely be acceptable for most uses.

Legal Nature of Labels

Though one out of every 100 Americans is statistically suffering from Celiac's, and the material acts as an irritant in the case of those with gluten intolerance, labels generally do not announce a product's gluten values as the FDA considers gluten to be a product GRAS (generally regarded as safe). Recent rulings do allow companies to promote a product voluntarily as being 'gluten-free' if they are provable to include less than 20 parts per million of the protein, a distinction that has medical as well as marketing merit.

Without considerably more stringent rulings, however, the best a consumer can do is be personally informed, and educate themselves further if the choice to live gluten-free is more than a simple lifestyle change, and their lives literally depend on being right about the substance. Read and study books like this one, so you are prepared.

When in Doubt, Do it Yourself.

Of course, beyond the prepared food alternatives and substitutions, there is always the exploration and wonder of making your own meals from scratch, from milling the kinds of grains that are allowed and making your own breads, pastas, and tortillas. Not only would such foods be clearly more natural and tasty, one could create one's own specialties, fine-tuning the process to perfection. There would be considerably more time invested in this way of avoiding gluten, but in the end, you would also be arguably healthier and wise to boot!

Such personalized cooking might even lend itself to a more social life, as there are others in the same situation, seeking to interconnect with others on the same kind of diet. The social aspects of this interconnection should not be overlooked; each person on this kind of crusade doesn't walk it alone, and there are much others can learn and teach along the way. And who knows, you might learn some new recipe ideas along the way.

4. The Other Reasons to Avoid Gluten

Perhaps you and your family are perfectly healthy, and don't have the issues that plague persons with Celiac's disease or other maladies. There seems to be a goodly sum of reasons that others seem to have come up with, for reducing or eliminating gluten from one's diet. This book would not be complete without covering these to some extent, to be a complete resource on the subject.

In this chapter, you will learn:

- The majority of reasons proponents give for taking on this dietary change, going so far as to become gluten free in their entire diet.

- Medical and professional opinions concerning the physical results of changing to a gluten-free lifestyle.

What the Proponents of Gluten-Free life offer

As one might expect, the proposed benefits of any dietary change includes weight loss and physical well-being. Further, and this is primarily anecdotal recommendations of those who had only been self-diagnosed, a whole raft of digestion-related maladies is suggested to have been remedied by removing gluten from one's diet. Bloating, indigestion, constipation, diarrhea, all are claimed to be resolved in those who claim sensitivity to gluten when they remove it from the diet.

There really is no definitive damage that is done when someone chooses to go gluten free, but there is still a danger of misunderstanding the hype, and considering products gluten-free that perhaps have other health dangers as a result. Many products that make the claim actually have more fats, more sugars, and generally do not have a healthful benefit; even some people who shifted to gluten-free gained weight instead!

When all is said and done, the only persons who truly benefit from a gluten-free diet are those who are health-conscious, and do suffer from some level of gluten sensitivity and intolerance. Be sure to confer with your doctor before any major dietary change, as is always the case.

What the Medical Profession and Experts have to say

Though it certainly benefits those particularly adversely impacted by intolerance and certain diseases, the medical community has not yet resoundingly supported a gluten-free diet. The reasons that there is not a lot of support for this train of thought stems first from the dietary good that gluten seems to have on normal digestion. Whole grains, like those that are main sources of the stuff, are well noted for aiding in reduced risk of heart disease, cancer, and even obesity and diabetes.

It is not sufficient to remove peanuts from consumption just because some folks have allergies. In fact, in most cases, gluten might even boost immune functions in those who do not suffer from Celaic's disease. In fact, the very presence of Gluten in one's diet can lead to discovery of their disease; if they have already started a gluten-free diet, the medical authorities might even miss a diagnosis of this, as the reaction to Gluten normally found as a trigger would be absent!

To further muddy the waters, there is mounting evidence that there may even be more going on than Gluten sensitivity in cases of Celiac's disease. So taking on a rigorous anti-gluten diet may not even be the best alternative for sufferers of this disease. In all cases, medical authorities should be consulted before any change of diet this extreme is undertaken.

Making Up Your Own Mind.

Despite all the hoopla from both the pro-gluten and the gluten-free viewpoints, the information that is out there is made available so you can make up your mind based on what others have said or done. There are support groups for Celiac's sufferers, those who are already walking the Gluten-Free path, and there are those who champion alternative treatments.

This book is only one resource; despite its concise and comprehensive coverage, other resources should be researched along the way to making up your mind about what you choose to do with your life. Talk to those who suffer from the disease, from those who suffer from the various levels of Gluten Intolerance and allergies. And most importantly, talk to your doctor and medical personnel. Make sure the decision is right for you.

5. Moderation in Dietary Experimentation

Diets are hard things to amend. We become familiar with certain foods, used to the taste and texture, and we learn how to prepare and gather those food items. So what happens, when we decide to make the major life changes that will save our lives, or even simply improve them? We make the attempt, stick with it a few days, then lapse back to our old habits.

Having talked exhaustively about what a Gluten-Free diet might entail, what can be said about getting relief from the symptoms that the Gluten-free approach claims to correct? What alternatives within this new gluten-awareness can be undertaken safely, with or without medical consultation?

In this chapter, you will learn:

- The dangers of extreme dietary change, and how to avoid them

- Several steps one can take to discover dietary balance without creating more trouble that it is worth.

A little change goes a long way

There may be small changes you can make to your diet, that will resolve the health issues you believe the gluten-free life might provide. Maybe you do have a bit of intolerance for one kind of gluten. such as for wheat, or perhaps you have difficulty digesting oats. Substituting one kind or type over a period of a few weeks might resolve your problem. The point is that many times our digestive system regulates itself with only minimal shifts on our part. Any number of causes can be in play that result in discomfort, or even symptoms of illness.

Rather than completely cutting gluten from your diet entirely, consider a hiatus, a short 'food vacation' from the major sources of gluten, to see if the there are any changes that result. As above, give the change a few weeks to manifest; your body does not change composition or dietary balance overnight, and there may be more variables at play than you might be considering.

Food-logs and subtlety

Whether or not you are looking for solutions to medical difficulties, tracking your actual food intake is an eye-opening experience for most people. In our rapid-fire world, often we don't think about what we take in, and because we are not even conscious of quantity and composition of our meals, snacks, and in-between treats, we can rack up a considerable arsenal of things that could contribute to our ill health.

By taking the time and the intent to track what we take in, ironically, we can alter our eating and digestion habits almost immediately. The sheer effort required to honestly list on paper what we eat, when we eat it, and even the circumstances that trigger our eating, we get a more realistic picture of our diet. One should track their eating, not just for a single day, but for several weeks, to identify trends and habits that can then by analyzed and considered for change. For your own satisfaction, be sure to track those primary sources of gluten you are eating. In doing so, you will either convince yourself that it might be a good idea to be screened for Celiac's disease – it is genetic, and finding out can not only help you, but your children or future children as well – or present you with other alternative causes of your health issues.

Consider all the options

While this booklet is aimed at the all-out Gluten-Free alternative, there are other viewpoints to consider. Talk to your medical advisers, and see if a restriction or limitation to Gluten would be advisable. Maybe going without glutens for a few days a month might be sufficient to manage your symptoms. Even two or three days a week might be more manageable, afford you enough freedom from symptoms to function.

Or perhaps there can be some directions as to which forms of glutens can be tolerated. Consider nutritional screenings, to see if more precise information can be gathered on which gluten types you are most susceptible to. There are more and deeper research projects going on all the time. Keep up with these projects, and remain informed.

Finally, there may be alternatives that can be put into place that might allow you to return to a diet with glutens, after your body recovers its resiliency. Again, medical professionals should be included in such decisions, but it might be one day possible to get away from a Gluten-Free lifestyle again at some point in the future.

6. Being Gluten Free on the Go

With all the emphasis on fast food, there are relatively few choices left to a person or family attempting to live gluten-free while traveling. Most fast-food restaurants focus on making food finger-friendly, meaning they wrap breads around most meal choices. We'll discuss some innovative alternatives that will keep your gluten-free when you aren't at home.

In this chapter, you will learn:

- Eating Opportunities and Options On the Go

- Quick Stop N Fix options 'Outside the Box'

Fast Food Alternatives

Burgers. Burritos. Even Pizza. All these options, so prevalent today, wrap good food in wrappers of gluten-clogged farinaceous breads, tortillas, and pizza dough. Fortunately, most of the fast food places have been made aware of this challenge, and nearly every one of them has at least one salad option. Granted, they might sneak some bread croutons into the mix, but with a little diligence on your part there are healthy alternatives around virtually every corner.

Grocery Grab and Go Options

Grocery stores, aware of the rapidly changing marketplace, have become wonderful servants of their communities. In most of them, there are now single-serving food options in the fruit and vegetable section, some with, and some without meat servings included. These are perfect for grabbing on the go, perhaps for a picnic in the park, or for those working lunches that employers seem to find so appealing these days. Just drop in, make your choice, and duck out through the express checkout lane. Easy, simple and fast.

All Around Healthy Fare for Any Time, Anywhere.

If we haven't belabored it enough already, the sources for gluten are relatively few and though also seemingly ubiquitous, easily avoidable, if you focus on fresh food, from meats, eggs, and cheese, to fruits and vegetables. Many communities now host farmer's markets, bringing just these types of foods together as a convenience and a social gathering. Add to this a few artisan bread makers who focus on the gluten-free aspect, and you have an instant resource that gives back every week!

7: Best Practices & Common Mistakes

As we have already cautioned, changing one's diet radically, even for the best of reasons, can be a dangerous business. Here are some tips when considering a transition to the trendy but perhaps not well-understood Gluten-Free lifestyle.

Do's

Consult your Physician

Your doctor will have the best information concerning your health, and he or she is as enthusiastic about good health as you are. So take the time, set an appointment, and talk candidly with them about what you are feeling, experiencing, and considering. Go over the health concerns you have, even your personal opinions about gluten and its effect on your body. Then, when the appropriate tests have been taken, they can best suggest a healthy course of action. It might be indeed that you have intolerances, or even suffer from Celiac's disease. In any case, it is always advisable to make dietary changes of this magnitude only under medical supervision.

Perform Due Diligence in Reading and Understanding Labeling

For a variety of reasons, food manufacturers and processors seek to use somewhat confusing labels when marking food regarding gluten and its inclusion. Become educated on what the various labels mean, and be sure to honestly evaluate the likelihood of the inclusion of Gluten in them. Some foods are surprisingly rife with the material, where others are completely devoid of it. By taking the time to know the difference you can accomplish your goals and stay healthy.

Be Certain of your True Agenda in Taking on a Gluten-Free Life.

Once you are certain that you are going to move to this kind of dietary limitation, do all you can to make the change completely. Remaining ignorant about gluten sources and the downside of including it in your diet can, in those extreme cases we have discussed, lead to extreme ill health, and perhaps worse. If your doctors have cleared you to change this extremely, only shift back with their awareness as well, because the sheer lack of gluten may have far-reaching ramifications for your health in other unseen ways.

Stay abreast of new developments.

Nothing remains the same for long. With all the research going on these days, it might be possible to adapt your lifestyle with new medications, rather than a restrictive diet in the future. You will want to keep abreast of the latest medical alternatives, and consider any medications that might arise. The medical professionals will help you to keep up with the alternatives.

Don'ts

Make dietary changes without medical input

While the fad and popularity votes call for radical lifestyle changes, your physician will certainly know better what is best for you. If you are concerned with the amount of gluten in your diet, wonder first what gave you that impression. If you have symptoms of gluten intolerance, check with your doctor. There are definitive tests for Celiac's disease, and if your doctor concurs, then you will be better informed as to how to proceed.

Trust the labels on food items, concerning the existence or volume of gluten.

Fads sell products, and while products often purport healthful attributes, the vagueness and unregulated way they advertise can be misleading. Take the tips you learned in this booklet, and be wary of any product that seems to suggest its lack of gluten. In particular, watch for the other things they may have amplified in order to do so - high sugar or fat content, even triglycerides and other unhealthful material. Be diligent and careful.

Take this or any dietary change lightly or frivolously.

For Celiac's disease sufferers, or even those with wheat or other intolerances, a shift in diet can mean life or death. If you are attracted to the concept of such healthful changes, it means your heart is in the right place, and making any positive healthy choices go a long way to bringing you improved health, and a better life overall. Just take care that your changes are not too abrupt or too zealous in their nature, that you endanger your overall health in favor of the fad-nature of such changes. Remember, it is your life and the quality thereof you are dealing with, and you would not want to risk a worse condition on a whim or fancy. Make your decisions with all the information at your fingertips, like this book and with your doctor's consent and advice.

Ignore or disregard the advice of your doctor.

Despite all the hype and recommendations of friends and colleagues, and regardless of all the positive press information on any given diet, one would do well to keep to the recommendations made by their doctor. Choosing to disregard or ignore such would be taking chances with your health, and put your life at risk. Be careful, and if you have any questions, do not hesitate to ask. That is their purpose.

Conclusion

Thank you for purchasing and reading this helpful handbook. As a guide we hope it has served to inform you about a Gluten-Free lifestyle, its value and challenges, and to give you the information you need to live a healthy life with or without gluten in your diet.

Our intent was to give you a guide to the Gluten-Free life, both with its positives and negatives, its proponents and detractors. In places, it may seem that this booklet pours cold water on the Gluten-Free lifestyle. In all candor, the choice to live gluten-free is yours to make, and in cases where medical recommendations accompany the decision, it is a very good one.

I have gone over the basics of the Gluten-free life, how difficult and challenging it is to seek out foods that are substitutes for the gluten-laden staples in the American diet. We addressed the various alternatives that could be used to mitigate the changes in eating habits. In those sections, we talked about dietary experimentation, and how tastes change over time, to accommodate the changes in the eating experience a little at a time.

I also covered the broad variety of labels that food producers use to alternately inform and confuse the consumer, and how very important it is that you perform your own investigation, and choose those foods that are truly gluten-free over those that claim to contain "less gluten" or "reduced gluten content", as these can be misleading.

In all, I have provided you with a coherent discussion of the Gluten-Free Lifestyle. Whether you pursue it as necessity, or choose to restrict Glutens in your diet for more personal reasons, you have everything you need to make an informed and educated effort.

I hope you find this booklet as useful and informative as it can be, and that you discover your own course in life taking advantage of its tips and information.

Thank you again for your purchase, and I hope this book is as helpful in guiding your lifestyle as it was enjoyable to write.

Just a friendly reminder. ☺

If you enjoyed this book, would you please leave a review for this book in the Kindle store? It'd be greatly appreciated!

Take a look at my other books:

HOW TO HAVE A SUCCESSFUL GARAGE SALE

SELLING GOODWILL ITEMS ON EBAY

Amazon Author Central Page

Facebook

Thanks Again

Sally Parker

www.ingramcontent.com/pod-product-compliance
Lightning Source LLC
Chambersburg PA
CBHW081139280526
45787CB00007B/3145

9781533001467